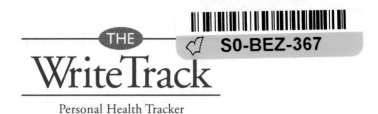

The WriteTrack

Personal Health Tracker

From my position on the examination table, I could see the ultrasound screen. The technician stopped the probe on an area. When I saw the asymmetrical shape of the "spot," I knew the diagnosis was breast cancer. The biopsy that immediately followed confirmed my suspicion. My mind raced, my chest ached, and I needed more information.

Research, knowledge, faith, prayers, and the support of family and friends were crucial to my treatment and recovery. One of the most valuable resources was *The WriteTrack* by Dr. Joe Wiederholt. For me, being informed and actively involved in the decisions regarding treatment was essential. Many sources provided the specifics, but documenting the symptoms and side effects was overwhelming. What did my doctor need to know? What side effects did I even remember between treatments? Because of the ease of use, organization, and design, I could record all of the information to share with my health care providers. Although I was unable to control the disease, I could cope by keeping "track."

The WriteTrack is a tremendous resource for cancer patients. It is a unique publication because it was developed by a medical professional who had cancer. Dr. Wiederholt's professional knowledge and personal perspectives allowed him to create a book that helps others.

Cancer treatment is an arduous journey, having a guidebook such as *The WriteTrack* is a blessing.

Anna—Breast Cancer Survivor

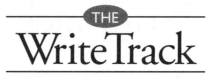

Personal Health Tracker

I was given a book by Joe Wiederholt, called *The WriteTrack*. It has been my guide to follow my treatment and well-being. I can track my progress with ease and it has helped with communication between my oncologist and me. Since my cancer diagnosis, I have had friends diagnosed with other cancers. I have recommended this book to them to help them organize all of the information that is thrown in their direction. The response has been unbelievable. They too, after being slapped in the face with this horrible disease, have had their lives made easier because of this book.

Mary Beth—Cancer Patient

As a nurse in the Cancer Center, I have found that patients who journal are able to provide their caregivers with more accurate histories of their symptoms throughout the chemotherapy process. This information in turn enables the clinicians to fine-tune the supportive care measures that are vital to the well-being of our patients. Patients love this journal. It is thoughtfully laid out and user-friendly. It helps them organize their appointments, document their symptoms, record their counts and express their feelings. It provides a sense of organization and control over an overwhelming situation.

Kathy Rothering, R.N.—Oncology Nurse

This little book was the best thing that we could have. I called it my "Bible." There are so many emotions and upheavals during this time. My "Bible" helped us track and keep all information together. Everyone should have this book.

Joseph and Wife—Cancer Patient and Spouse

The clients I work with tell me that *The WriteTrack* was an invaluable tool which helped them organize information, document their experiences and perceptions, and then retrieve what they needed as their treatment progressed. I believe *The WriteTrack* helps our clients comprehend and absorb the oftentimes frightening and complex world of cancer treatment and survivorship.

Neil J. O'Connor, ACSW, LCSW—Senior Clinical Social Worker

THE WriteTrack

Personal Health Tracker for Cancer Patients

NEW EDITION

by Joe Wiederholt
with Peggy Wiederholt

About the cover:
The Katsura Tree on the cover has been named in memory of the author, Joe
Wiederholt. Located in the University of Wisconsin Arboretum, Joe found refuge on a
bench under the tree throughout his cancer journey. The heart-shaped leaves represent
both his deep appreciation of nature and his inspiring love of life.

Published by Wiederholt Group, Inc.
www.thewritetrack.net

Distributed by Goblin Fern Press, Inc.
Toll-free: 888-670-2665

ISBN-10: 0-9771847-0-6
ISBN-13: 978-0-9771847-0-5
LCCN: 2005909199

To order more copies or for quantity discounts, go to www.thewritetrack.net

A portion of the proceeds from this book will be donated to cancer research.

Printed in the United States
First Printing

Dedication

*To the memory of Joe Wiederholt,
loving husband, devoted father,
and teacher to all who knew him.*

1949—2001

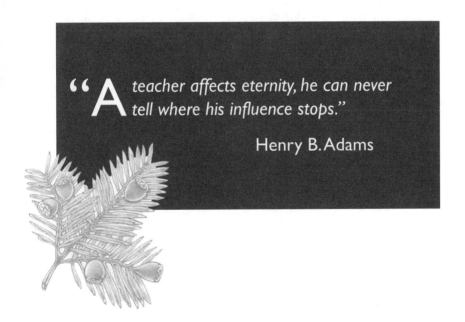

" **A** *teacher affects eternity, he can never
tell where his influence stops.*"

Henry B. Adams

Acknowledgements

Joe was the creative force behind the development of *The WriteTrack* from the time he initially thought of the idea in 1994, during his own cancer journey, until the book was first published in 1997. His spirit has continued to be the motivation for subsequent editions. However, he would be the first to join me in acknowledging the contributions of so many others who were involved in the creative process.

Our children, Jade Wiederholt and Mekel Wiederholt Meier, are our greatest source of inspiration. They make life worth living.

Cancer patients who have used and critiqued this book are truly the greatest contributors. Their suggestions have made this a better, more useful tool.

Gabe Leung, former senior marketing director at Bristol-Myers Squibb Company (BMS), believed in Joe's idea. BMS provided support and funding for the first version of *The WriteTrack* in 1997 and again in 2001, making it available to thousands of cancer patients nationally.

Susan Eno Collins, Diane Teasdale and Roy Broadfoot at HealthEd (formerly Doctors + Designers), embraced the project and collaborated with Joe to develop his idea into a book. Their personal commitment was clearly demonstrated by the publication of a commemorative edition of *The WriteTrack* in 2002 following Joe's death.

Carol Hermanson-Dobulnicky, Ph.D. University of Wyoming, and Betty Chewning, Ph.D., University of Wisconsin, investigated the positive impact of having cancer patients use the self-monitoring calendars contained within *The WriteTrack* in a clinical trial at the University of Wisconsin Comprehensive Cancer Center. Both Carol and Betty continue to use *The WriteTrack* in their research and teaching, and in national and international scholarly presentations and publications.

Howard Bailey, M.D., University of Wisconsin Comprehensive Cancer Center, was Joe's medical oncologist and our health care partner. Howard understood the importance of patient-provider communication and shared decision making. His compassion, willingness to listen, and support for patients, make him a true role model for health care providers.

Kira Henschel, Goblin Fern Press, Inc., has provided both guidance and support. Her knowledge and ability to encourage and motivate have been priceless.

Sincere thanks to you all!

Peggy Wiederholt

INSIDE *The Write Track*

Foreword...

Preface...

Introduction...

Welcome to *The Write Track*...

Your Personal Records...

Finding Support...

Personal Planner...

Important Telephone Contacts and Numbers

Personal Thoughts

FOREWORD

My husband, Dan, was diagnosed with colorectal cancer in 1993. Unlike Dr. Joe Wiederholt, and his wife, Peggy, he did not have a plan to fight his disease and a plan to live his life to the fullest in the time he had.

If he had, it might not have made a difference.

His time was very short, and most spent in trying to feel comfort for just one day.

Dan lived only four months from his diagnosis until his death, leaving behind his wife and three young sons, as well as a daughter from his previous marriage, and his siblings-one of whom would live only one more year after him-and many beloved friends.

Joe Wiederholt's courageous and conscious battle did not end in victory over cancer, either, but it did end in a victory over the dark. He managed his life, his treatment, and his understanding of his treatment in this valley of shadow with grace and dignity. His wife, Peggy, continued his work and is publishing the new edition of *The WriteTrack*, a journal and planning tool for cancer patients, so that others can follow the inspiring journey he pioneered.

I met Peggy when I was working to make people aware of colorectal cancer and the hope that now exists for extending the life of people even with end stage disease. Her story and her hard work were so inspiring-both for the many who now survive and thrive after cancer and those who do not. She was determined to empower others, and to honor her husband in the process.

Please give *The WriteTrack* to anyone who knows someone who has cancer, is living with someone who has cancer, who treats people with cancer, or works with people who have cancer. It is a powerful work of substance and faith.

Jacquelyn Mitchard
Best-selling author and cancer prevention advocate

national conferences and with pharmacy students in the classroom, emphasizing the importance of monitoring side effects and improving communication between healthcare professionals and patients, being a real patient advocate.

Joe was also convinced that a side effect tracking system like the one he had used for himself could help other chemotherapy patients. The very thought of it energized and excited him. His enthusiasm soon became contagious. He contacted a former graduate student who was in the Oncology Division of Bristol-Myers Squibb Company and shared his idea. The idea was quickly embraced and HealthEd (formerly Doctors + Designers), a company with expertise in developing patient-centered health education materials, was soon involved. The project also received the support and approval of Cancer Care, Inc. Working as a team, they were able to take Joe's one-page side effect monitoring diary and develop it into *The Write Track.*

After a year of chemotherapy, Joe's cancer was in remission until the fall of 1999, when he was diagnosed with metastatic disease. He used *The Write Track* to monitor the side effects of chemotherapy regimens and eventually radiation therapy as well. He gained much satisfaction from knowing that perhaps he played a role in helping other cancer patients cope with their disease. When interviewed by a local television station after being honored with a national teaching award, the reporter commented on how Joe's experience with cancer seemed to have some positive effects on his life. Joe smiled broadly and said, "The neatest thing I had happen when I started therapy the second time was … I sat in the clinic, people didn't know who I was, and a patient pulled out *The Write Track.* That was … WOW!"

Joe's life ended on May 28, 2001; however his legacy of helping patients through his research and teaching continues. Research based on *The Write Track* has been presented at national and international scientific conferences and has been published in scientific journals.

Joe's dream was to make *The Write Track* available to any cancer patient who wishes to use it. Since it was first published in 1997, over 150,000 copies have been printed. This newly revised version incorporates helpful suggestions made by cancer patients and health care providers who have used previous editions.

I have experienced using *The Write Track* both as an oncology nurse and as the wife of a cancer patient. In addition, when Joe was undergoing cancer treatments, one of his caregivers was my mother, Dorothy Feeley. He lovingly called her "Nurse #2." Diagnosed with lung cancer in May of 2005, Nurse #2 has reminded our family yet again of the value of this book on a very personal level. It is our hope that *The Write Track* will help you on your cancer journey.

1. Quote from: Wiederholt JB, Wiederholt P. "The patient! Our teacher and friend." *American Journal of Pharmaceutical Education.* 1997;61.

"What lies behind us and lies before us are tiny matters compared to what lies within us."

Ralph Waldo Emerson

The WriteTrack

"**O**nce my doctors told me I had cancer, my mind traveled at warp speed. One second I'd think about my job...the next my wife...the next our children...the next my mom and dad, brothers and sisters, other relatives...the next life in general...the next death. When traveling at warp speed, the content of my thoughts followed no particular pattern. Tracking my experiences in a calendar helped me gain some control and cope with it."

Joe Wiederholt

Welcome to *The WriteTrack*

The WriteTrack is a personal health tracker developed specifically for people who are undergoing chemotherapy and/or radiation treatment for cancer. What's unique about *The WriteTrack* is that the calendars, tracking charts, and information are based on first-hand experiences and personal insights of cancer survivors.

During the development of *The WriteTrack*, people with cancer openly shared information and tips they found most helpful in getting through their treatments as comfortably as possible. Many people found the days seemed to blur together and it was often hard to remember details. Keeping personal calendars throughout treatment helped these cancer survivors keep track of important information and cope better with treatment.

Track your treatment...and more

In *The WriteTrack*, you will find monthly and weekly calendars to track...

cx Your treatment schedule

cx Appointments

cx Symptoms of cancer

cx Side effects of treatment

The WriteTrack also offers ideas to help you get ready for visits to your health care team, recognize symptoms and side effects, and learn how to ask for help from family and friends.

Everyone has individual needs and will use *The WriteTrack* differently. Not everyone will want to record information about their treatment. If this is true for you, consider sharing *The WriteTrack* with a close family member or trusted friend who may want to do the recording for you.

There is only one rule when using *The WriteTrack*—that is to use it how you want. *The WriteTrack* is your personal calendar. It is designed so you can easily adjust it to your needs. You may find some sections more helpful to you than others—feel free to use only those sections you find most helpful.

While using *The WriteTrack*, you may also find the type and amount of information you want to track will change over time. You may even choose to track information for a while, then take a break. Just remember that however you use *The WriteTrack* is your choice.

The information that follows is brief—it is only intended to give a starting place from which you, your family, and friends can learn more. Some valuable resources and organizations are also included. It is important to remember the information contained in *The WriteTrack* is not intended and should not be used as a substitute for advice or information from your health care team. Please talk to your health care team if you have any questions about cancer and your treatment.

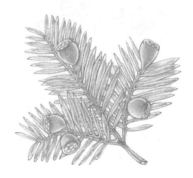

"If I had one piece of advice for someone going through cancer treatment, I would tell them, 'Get as much information as you can.' Being informed makes you feel more in control...more prepared, and less anxious. But don't get all the information at once...get information at each stage of your treatment. When I was diagnosed, I wanted to learn what the types and stages of cancer meant. When I was deciding on treatment, I wanted to know the pros and cons of treatment options. When I was beginning treatment, I wanted to know what side effects I could expect.

Think of getting information like eating 10 dinners...you would never eat all 10 dinners in one day. You would spread the dinners out. It's the same with information... break it into small parts so you can digest what's important to you."

Denise
Thyroid Cancer Survivor

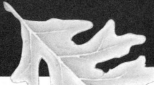

Information is a powerful tool. It can give you a sense of control, which is very important as you continue through cancer treatment. Yet, don't feel you have to know and learn everything all at once—this could leave you feeling overwhelmed and afraid. In fact, it is often better to gather as much information as you want, then sort it by topics, and use it as you need it.

> "There was great depth...and meaning in my wife's role as I went through treatment—words can't express how important she was to me. She was an advocate for me in so many ways... including being my information buddy.
>
> I had stacks and stacks of information on cancer and its treatment. I didn't know where to start reading...my wife helped me sort the piles so I could focus on what information was really relevant to me at the time."
>
> Joe Wiederholt

Recruit an information buddy

You may want to consider asking a family member or friend you trust, someone who knows you very well, to be your information buddy. An information buddy can help you gather and sort information on each aspect of your treatment and care and provide it to you as you need it. This person should also be someone who is persistent and assertive—that way you will know you can count on them to get the information you need, when you need it.

At first, you may find that family and friends are uncomfortable talking about your diagnosis of cancer and its treatment. It may help if you start the discussion by talking to them about your need for an information buddy.

Making informed decisions about treatment

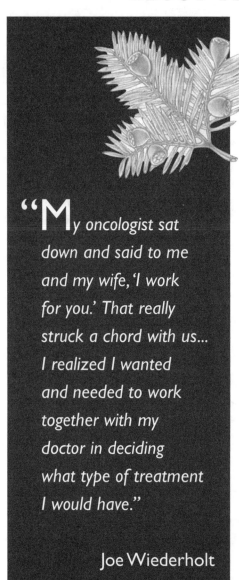

The decision to undergo treatment for cancer is individual. There are many considerations for you and your health care team to take into account, including:

- The type of cancer you have.

- What stage the cancer is in or how far it has progressed.

- Your age.

- Your physical well-being.

- Any other medical conditions you may have.

- Your personal needs and values.

What are clinical trials?

Clinical trials are research studies conducted with people who volunteer to participate. They are designed to answer scientific questions and to find new and better ways to prevent, diagnose and treat diseases.

Taking part in a clinical trial may be an opportunity to receive a new treatment not yet available to other cancer patients or to receive standard treatments in a new way. To learn more, ask your doctor or contact the National Cancer Institute (NCI) at www.cancer.gov or call the Cancer Information Service at 1-800-4-CANCER (1-800-422-6237).

"My oncologist sat down and said to me and my wife, 'I work for you.' That really struck a chord with us... I realized I wanted and needed to work together with my doctor in deciding what type of treatment I would have."

Joe Wiederholt

How to make informed decisions

Use the following questions as a guide when discussing and planning your treatment with your health care team. You may also want to get help from your information buddy. Sometimes it may be easier for them to ask questions and get answers. By asking these questions and getting answers you understand, you can make informed decisions...and take an active role in your treatment. Asking these questions may naturally lead to other important questions that will also help you make decisions.

Ꮗ What types of treatment are available to you?

Ꮗ What is involved with each of these treatments?

Ꮗ Which treatment is recommended for you?

Ꮗ Why is this treatment recommended?

Ꮗ What are the goals of this treatment?

Ꮗ How does this cancer treatment work?

Ꮗ What realistic expectations should you have about this treatment?

Ꮗ What types of medicine, if any, will be used with this treatment?

Ꮗ Why will these medicines be used?

Ꮗ Are there any specific side effects you may experience as a result of the medicines and treatment?

Ꮗ What are the risks and benefits of not getting treatment?

Getting a second opinion...

You may wish to get a second opinion before deciding on a treatment. This is common, so most doctors are comfortable with this request and often help you with a referral. Be sure to check with your insurance company first, however, to find out what your policy covers. You can also contact the American Cancer Society for information on getting another opinion at 800-ACS-2345 or www.cancer.org.

After you have made a decision, use pages 8 and 9 to record important information about your treatment plan.

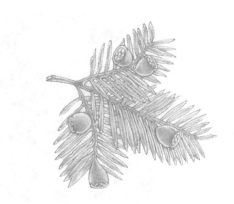

TREATMENT PLAN

Use this page to write down information about your cancer and the treatment plan.

Make sure all of your questions are answered before you begin treatment.

Type of Cancer:

My Treatment Plan:

_____

_____

_____

_____

_____

_____

_____

_____

_____

_____

_____

_____

> "The richness of the human experience would lose something of rewarding joy if there were no limitations to overcome."
>
> Helen Keller

TREATMENT GUIDELINES

Your health care team may provide you with certain guidelines and precautions that should be followed during treatment. For example, if you are treated with radiation therapy, instructions on proper skin care are very important. This page can be used to record special instructions and other information that you find helpful as you start your treatments.

> **"O**ften patients feel they have to 'follow orders'...
> instead, patients should work with their health care team
> to set up a treatment schedule that takes into account
> their needs...and what's important to them. Getting
> involved...can give patients that important sense of control."
>
> Carol
> *Oncology Nurse*

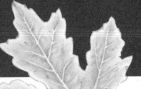

Help plan your schedule

Once you decide on a treatment plan (also called a treatment protocol), the next step is to set up a treatment schedule—that is, the days and times you will receive treatment. Work together with your health care team to plan your schedule. You may want to ask your information buddy to be a part of this as well. When planning your schedule, find out if there is room for flexibility. Flexibility in the schedule may vary depending on the treatment site and the equipment available. It is important to know that your schedule is not always etched in stone, so talk to your health care team.

As you plan your schedule, also state your concerns, needs, and priorities to your health care team. Start by asking yourself these questions...

What about upcoming activities?

Are there any holidays or important social engagements you really want to be able to attend?

What days and what time of day will be best for you to get the treatment?

What days and what time of day will be easiest for a family member or friend to go along with you?

When planning your treatment schedule, also ask these questions...

Who will give you the treatment?
Know which members of your health care team will be present at each treatment. Also know what their role is in your treatment.

Will you see the oncologist at each treatment?

You may not always see your oncologist. Knowing ahead of time whether or not your oncologist will be present can help put you at ease.

Can you and should you bring a family member or friend to each treatment?

You may find it very comforting to have a family member or friend with you. Be sure to ask if you can have someone with you while getting treatment.

Will you need someone to drive you home after treatment?

Find out if you will need a driver so you can make arrangements. Your information buddy may be able to help you.

Will you need to stay in the hospital or in bed for any length of time following treatment?

Knowing if this is a possibility can help you plan ahead and be prepared.

Is your schedule flexible once it is set up?

As you keep track of your treatments in the weekly and monthly calendars and monitor how you feel in the days following treatment, you may be able to spot certain trends and predict the days you will feel good. If your schedule has any flexibility, you may be able to adjust it slightly so you know you will feel good on the days that are most important to you.

> "*It's my body...so I wanted the oncologist to tell me what was going to happen during chemotherapy. Being informed let me be an active partner in my care.*"
>
> Lisa
> *Breast Cancer Survivor*

Know what to expect

As you plan your treatment schedule, also ask what to expect with treatment. This will help make you feel less anxious and more comfortable. People who have been through treatment suggest you ask your health care team to...

- "Walk you" through the treatment.

- Tell you about the sights, sounds, and smells you can expect.

- Describe what getting the treatment will feel like.

- Describe how you might feel right after treatment and in the hours and days following treatment.

Know your health care team

It is likely that you will have a number of medical professionals on your health care team. Some of them may include...

Dietitian—a health care provider who guides people in planning their food choices to ensure they get proper nutrition. The dietitian is an excellent resource for helping people going through treatment for cancer cope with appetite and weight problems, if they occur.

Medical oncologist—a doctor who specializes in the administration of a variety of medicines needed to treat cancer.

Oncology nurse—a nurse who is trained to care for people going through treatment of cancer. An oncology nurse will carry out the treatment plan determined by you and your health care team. In addition to coordinating your care, oncology nurses give medicines; monitor symptoms and side effects; and can provide information, tips, and advice as you go through treatment.

Pharmacist—a medical professional who is trained to prepare and dispense medicine. A pharmacist can monitor your treatment with respect to cancer medicines and medicines you may be taking for other medical conditions or diseases. A pharmacist is an excellent resource for learning more about your medicines.

Physical therapist—a medical professional who is trained in the use of physical treatments, such as exercise and massage.

Radiation oncologist—a doctor who specializes in the use of radiation to treat cancer.

Radiation therapist—a medical professional who is trained to run the equipment that delivers the radiation treatment.

Radiologist—a medical professional who is trained to read and explain diagnostic x-rays of areas inside your body and perform specialized x-ray procedures.

Social worker—a professional who is trained to provide counseling and practical assistance to meet your specific needs. The social worker can provide counseling to help you cope with concerns and issues related to diagnosis, treatment, symptoms, and side effects of cancer. Individual, family, and support group counseling can be offered.

The WriteTrack can help

Refer to the Important Telephone Numbers section of *The WriteTrack* (see pages 160-161) and record...

cs The names of every professional on your health care team.

cs Their role in your treatment.

cs Their telephone numbers and extensions, along with the hours when they can be reached.

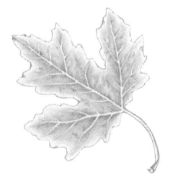

TREATMENT SCHEDULE

Cancer survivors have expressed how helpful it was to write out their complete treatment schedule so they could see the whole timeline in front of them. They also used the timeline as a countdown to their last treatment. If you think this will be helpful to you, use the chart that follows.

In addition to recording in the chart the treatment numbers, dates, and times, you may also want to record the type of treatment you will receive. Use the "Type of treatment" column to note whether you will receive radiation, chemotherapy or another type of treatment. Record the information that will be most helpful to you—for example, if you are to receive chemotherapy, consider writing the names of specific chemotherapy medicines you will receive each time.

Keep in mind that your treatment schedule may not be written in stone. Along the way, it may be necessary for you or your health care team to make a few changes.

Treatment number	Date/Time	Type of treatment	Notes

Treatment number	Date/Time	Type of treatment	Notes

Treatment number	Date/Time	Type of treatment	Notes

Finding ways to cope with symptoms and side effects

> "As I was about to start treatment, I had major questions...How would it feel?...How are my body and mind going to adjust to it?...How could I learn ways to cope with it and have some sense of control?"
>
> Joe Wiederholt

The role of your health care team is not only to help you choose the best treatment available to fight your cancer — it is also to work with you to help you get through the entire treatment as comfortably as possible.

Share information

Depending on your specific situation, there will be a number of ways to manage any symptoms and side effects you may experience. To begin finding ways to cope, share information with your health care team—especially your oncologist, nurse, dietitian, and social worker. Take advantage of their knowledge and expertise. Your health care team can give you information, tips, and suggestions they have learned over years of working closely with others who have been through similar experiences. Also, talk openly and honestly about any symptoms or side effects you experience. Often, people believe they have to "live with the pain" or "tough it out". This is not true— you have the right to have your symptoms and side effects controlled. Your health care team can help.

Prepare for possible side effects

Before treatment begins, talk to your health care team about any possible side effects you may experience. Knowing this in advance can help you be prepared. For example, some people will have a loss of appetite and weight throughout treatment. If appetite and weight loss are a problem for you, talk to your health care team. Sometimes medication can be prescribed to help. Also talk to the dietitian on your team about developing an eating plan that is right for you.

Another possible side effect to talk to your health care team about is hair loss. Ask your oncologist and others on your health care team if hair loss is a side effect you can expect to experience. If it is, also find out how long after treatment starts you might begin losing your hair and if it is likely your hair will grow back when treatment is over.

Hair loss is often a sensitive issue. Cancer survivors have offered suggestions to help prepare for hair loss. You can find these on the next page. Keep in mind some of the suggestions may work for you, while others may not.

> "I was devastated when my hair fell out...it made having cancer seem so visible to me, my family, friends, and even strangers. Not having hair made me feel so blue...then I began to meet others who had lost their hair from treatment...their hair grew back thicker and stronger. This seemed symbolic to me... after treatment my hair, my body, and my soul would be stronger."
>
> Sally
> Breast Cancer Survivor

Coping with hair loss

- Consider sporting a new, shorter hairstyle—that way it may not seem like so much hair is falling out. Some cancer survivors also suggested considering the possibility of shaving your head before treatment begins. Again, this may or may not be an option for you.

- Think about what will make you feel most comfortable — maybe it's wearing a wig or hairpiece...wearing hats or scarves...or perhaps it's wearing nothing at all on your head.

- Wear sunscreen with a sun protection factor (SPF) of at least 15 to protect your scalp from the harmful effects of the sun and burning if you choose not to cover your head. Use SPF 45 if you are undergoing radiation treatment.

- If you want to wear a wig or hairpiece, try to buy it before treatment begins—that way you can match the color and texture to your natural hair.

- Some people who had always thought about trying different hairstyles or colors and never did, found this to be a good time to experiment.

- Wigs and hairpieces are tax deductible medical expenses, so keep your receipts. Also check with your health insurance provider— these expenses may be covered by your plan.

- At night, you may want to wear a soft cotton knit cap. It can help keep you warm and comfortable.

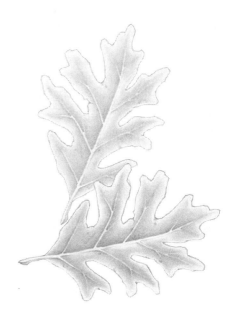

Valuable resources for coping with side effects

Look Good...Feel Better

This innovative workshop was developed by the Cosmetic, Toiletry, and Fragrance Association in cooperation with the American Cancer Society. It focuses on ways to help people undergoing cancer treatment enhance their appearance and feel better about themselves. Visit them at www.lookgoodfeelbetter.org or call for a list of local workshops.

800-395-LOOK
(800-395-5665)

Radiation Therapy and You: A Guide to Self-Help During Treatment

Chemotherapy and You: A Guide to Self-Help During Treatment

Eating Hints for Cancer Patients

These helpful and practical guides provide information on what to expect from chemotherapy and/or radiation treatment. Each guide offers useful tips for managing potential side effects of treatment, as well as many food and eating tips and recipes.

Available from the
National Cancer Institute
800-4-CANCER
(800-422-6237)

Caring for the Patient With Cancer at Home: A Guide for Patients and Families

This is an easy-to-read, practical guidebook for managing symptoms and side effects of cancer and its treatment. The book tells you what to do, what not to do, and gives guidance on when you should call for help from your health care team.

Available from the
American Cancer Society
800-ACS-2345
(800-227-2345)

Patients, Families and Friends... Cancer Reference Information

The American Cancer Society website provides numerous resources for patients, their families and friends.

Visit them at www.cancer.org.

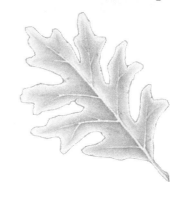

> **"I** thought about what activities I really enjoyed...which activities really made me feel good. The things I usually did on weekends with my wife and children were the most important...so on the days between treatments, when I felt good, I focused on doing fun things with my family."
>
> Joe Wiederholt

As you go through treatment, you'll find there are days you feel lousy or "low". On the brighter side, there will be days that you feel good and have plenty of energy. There's no doubt that you will want to take advantage of your better days and do things that you may have been putting off.

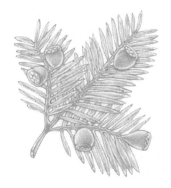

How to get the most out of your good days

- Think about doing the activities that you really value—the things that make you happy and lift your spirits, such as your favorite hobby, going for walks or being with family and friends.

- Schedule your favorite activities for the days you think you will be feeling good. *The WriteTrack* can help you predict these days.

- Plan to do some activities by yourself especially if you are wanting to feel independent. This can really help boost your confidence and morale.

- Think quality, not quantity. Rather than cram your good days full of activities and risk feeling tired, worn out, and frustrated the next day, prioritize what's most important to you. Take time to enjoy a few activities rather than overdoing it.

- Take rests or naps as you need them. This will help you recover your energy.

- Feel good about doing what is most important to you and what gives you pleasure. Just because you are having a good day and have a lot of energy, doesn't mean you have to spend the day doing household chores or running errands. This could leave you feeling run down or tired. You can choose to ask family and friends for support. In many cases they will be more than willing to help. In fact, helping you will probably make them feel really good. Turn to page 134 for advice about Getting Support From Family & Friends.

> "At least once a week...take time to really pamper yourself. Do something special just for you...as a way to congratulate yourself for going through another week of treatment."
>
> Denise
> Thyroid Cancer Survivor

The following calendar pages provide a way for you to capture important information one week at a time. One of the highlights of the weekly calendars is symptoms and side effects tracking. Many people who went through cancer treatment found it very helpful to record and track this information. It helped them recognize trends or patterns that developed between treatments and find ways to be more comfortable. Use the weekly calendars as you want. To help you get the most out of them, you may want to...

Record and track symptoms

Symptoms are signs of a disease, such as cancer. They are the effects of the disease on your body. Some examples of symptoms include unusual bleeding, a lump, hoarseness, and pain. Depending on the type of cancer, symptoms and how severe they are can vary from one person to another. Talk to your health care team about your symptoms. With today's advances in cancer care, many symptoms—especially pain—can be controlled.

"Being diagnosed with cancer made me feel like my life was spinning out of control...When I started chemotherapy, I kept a calendar and tracked how my body felt from one day to the next. I started to see certain trends. I could plan each day accordingly since I was able to predict my 'good' days and 'not-so-good' days. It also gave me a lot more information to share with my doctor. This helped me stay with my treatment and it gave me a tremendous sense of control."

Joe Wiederholt

...and side effects

Side effects sometimes occur as a result of taking medicine to treat cancer or having chemotherapy or radiation treatment. Some examples of side effects include nausea, appetite and weight loss, diarrhea, constipation, hair loss, and a tingling sensation in fingers or toes. Some people will experience side effects, while others may not. Among those who do experience them, the specific side effects and how severe they are can vary. If you do have side effects, let your health care team know. There are ways to help control them and make you feel more comfortable.

> **"M**y nurse always asked me if I was feeling fatigued...that wasn't what I would call how I felt...I just knew I had some days when my body felt completely zapped."
>
> Joe Wiederholt

Use your own words

You may want to use the weekly or monthly calendar pages of *The WriteTrack* to record how you feel physically and emotionally. When describing how you feel, don't worry about using medical terms—simply use your own words. Try to share this valuable information with your health care team.

Be honest about how you feel

When describing how you feel, be honest. When your health care team asks how you are feeling and what has been happening since your last visit or treatment, be specific rather than saying "OK", "not so good..." or "really good". Describe anything unusual to you—even if it seems unimportant. For instance, you might say something like, "I've had more energy over the last few days, but the pain got worse three days after my last treatment." Information like this can go a long way in helping your health care team help you. When it comes to dealing with symptoms or side effects such as pain, remember you don't have to "just live with them". Your health care team is there to work with you to control pain and any other symptoms or side effects you might have. To get the best help possible, they must first know how you honestly feel.

Let's take a look at how one person undergoing treatment chose to use the weekly calendar. This is the page from his first week of treatment.

1 Fill in the days and dates of the week →

Week of: 10/27 - 11/2

First week of therapy

Monday

Chemo - 2 drugs
Took med for nausea

Tuesday

Chemo - 1 drug
Took med for nausea
Took pain med

Wednesday

Chemo - 1 drug
Took med for nausea
Took pain med

Thursday

Chemo - 1 drug
Jan & Eric to stop by to watch a movie

Friday

No chemo
Bill's birthday

Saturday

No chemo
Not in the mood to eat, no appetite

Sunday

No chemo
Family picnic

30

2 **Rate and track your symptoms and side effects**

| mptoms and side effects | | | | 0 1 2 3 4 5 6 7 8 9 10
none low mild medium high | | | |

Day/date	10/27	10/28	10/29	10/30	10/31	11/1	11/2
Nausea	2	3	1	0			
ppetite loss						7	4
Diarrhea							
onstipation							
Pain		5	2	1			
Fatigue			2	2	2		
Tingling in feet/toes							
hing		2	3	4	4	4	4
amping	1	1	2	2	2	3	2
ange in ell	1	2	5	6	6	6	6

3 **Rate how severe symptoms and side effects are for you each day (see page 29)**

onal notes:

have had these weird changes in my sense of smell
my body itches - I have to ask the doctor about that!

the doctor's office this week, I struck up a
versation with a couple of people in the waiting
m - we had a few laughs... listening to them made
start to realize I am not alone.

appetite is not so good - have lost a couple of
nds. Will talk to the doctor.

4 **Jot down questions... plus personal thoughts and feelings**

The *WriteTrack* Weekly Calendar consists of four main sections you can use as you want to fit your needs. Let's take a look at how you might use each of these sections.

> **Week of:** 10/27
> First week of therapy
> Monday
> Chemo - 2 drugs
> Took med for nausea

Symptoms and side effects			
Day/date	10/27	10/28	10/2:
Nausea	2	3	1
Appetite loss			
Diarrhea			

1 Fill in the days and dates of the week

For each week, fill in the correct days and dates. Use this to help you track health care appointments; treatment days and times; business meetings; social activities; special dates to remember; how you feel that day; or anything else that is important to you.

2 Track your symptoms and side effects

You may want to track symptoms and side effects every day or you may prefer to reflect back on the entire week—then record what stands out. To help you get started, some examples of symptoms and side effects are shown. You may or may not experience these. Blank spaces are also provided for you to fill in any other symptoms or side effects you want to track. Don't feel you have to fill in each blank space.

It's important to create a list using your own words. Remember, over time your list may change if you want to track different symptoms and side effects. You may even want to take breaks from tracking once you learn the trends, how they relate to your treatment, and what can be done to help you feel more comfortable.

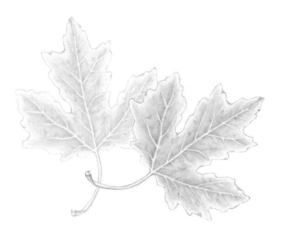

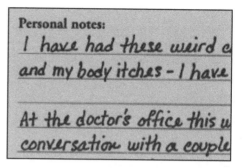

effects

| | 10/28 | 10/29 | 10/30 | 10/31 |
| 7 | 3 | 1 | 0 | |

Personal notes:

I have had these weird c
and my body itches - I have

At the doctor's office this u
conversation with a couple

3 Rate your symptoms and side effects

By rating how severe your symptoms and side effects are from week to week, you may spot certain trends that develop. You may also learn to recognize how the side effects relate to the day of your treatment; if there are trends with medicine you might be taking; how active you are from one day to the next; or how certain foods affect you. All of this can help you and your health care team find ways to cope with symptoms and side effects.

Consider using this scale to rate how severe your symptoms and side effects are:

| 0 | 1 2 | 3 4 5 | 6 7 8 | 9 10 |
| none | low | mild | medium | high |

You can also make up your own scale using other numbers or symbols.

4 Jot down questions...plus personal thoughts and feelings

Use the blank space on each page of the weekly calendar to write down any questions you want to ask your health care team. It's a good idea to write them down as they come to mind. That way you will be able to remember your important questions. These questions can also be recorded in the Health Care Visits section of *The WriteTrack* (see pages 94-119). The blank space can also be used to write down your thoughts and feelings. You may even want to try doodling or drawing pictures of how you feel. If you need more space, turn to pages 163-173.

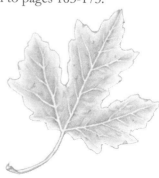

Week of:

Symptoms and side effects tracking

Day/date
 ———— ———— ———— ———— ———— ———— ————

Nausea

Appetite loss

Diarrhea

Constipation

Pain

Fatigue

Tingling in
fingers/toes

Depression

Personal notes:

Week of:

Symptoms and side effects tracking

0	1 2	3 4 5	6 7 8	9 10
none	low	mild	medium	high

Day/date ——— ——— ——— ——— ——— ——— ———

Nausea

Appetite loss

Diarrhea

Constipation

Pain

Fatigue

Tingling in
fingers/toes

Depression

_____

_____

_____

Personal notes:

Symptoms and side effects tracking

Day/date   ——   ——   ——   ——   ——   ——   ——

Nausea   ——   ——   ——   ——   ——   ——   ——

Appetite loss   ——   ——   ——   ——   ——   ——   ——

Diarrhea   ——   ——   ——   ——   ——   ——   ——

Constipation   ——   ——   ——   ——   ——   ——   ——

Pain   ——   ——   ——   ——   ——   ——   ——

Fatigue   ——   ——   ——   ——   ——   ——   ——

Tingling in
fingers/toes   ——   ——   ——   ——   ——   ——   ——

Depression   ——   ——   ——   ——   ——   ——   ——

——————   ——   ——   ——   ——   ——   ——

——————   ——   ——   ——   ——   ——   ——

——————   ——   ——   ——   ——   ——   ——

Personal notes:

Week of:

Symptoms and side effects tracking

0	1 2	3 4 5	6 7 8	9 10
none	low	mild	medium	high

Day/date	———	———	———	———	———	———	———
Nausea							
Appetite loss							
Diarrhea							
Constipation							
Pain							
Fatigue							
Tingling in fingers/toes							
Depression							
———							
———							
———							

Personal notes:

Week of:

Symptoms and side effects tracking

0	1 2	3 4 5	6 7 8	9 10
none	low	mild	medium	high

Day/date	——	——	——	——	——	——	——
Nausea							
Appetite loss							
Diarrhea							
Constipation							
Pain							
Fatigue							
Tingling in fingers/toes							
Depression							

Personal notes:

Week of: _____

Symptoms and side effects tracking

Day/date	——	——	——	——	——	——	——
Nausea	——	——	——	——	——	——	——
Appetite loss	——	——	——	——	——	——	——
Diarrhea	——	——	——	——	——	——	——
Constipation	——	——	——	——	——	——	——
Pain	——	——	——	——	——	——	——
Fatigue	——	——	——	——	——	——	——
Tingling in fingers/toes	——	——	——	——	——	——	——
Depression	——	——	——	——	——	——	——
————	——	——	——	——	——	——	——
————	——	——	——	——	——	——	——
————	——	——	——	——	——	——	——

Personal notes:

Week of:

Symptoms and side effects tracking

	0	1 2	3 4 5	6 7 8	9 10
	none	low	mild	medium	high

Day/date ——— ——— ——— ——— ——— ——— ———

Nausea							
Appetite loss							
Diarrhea							
Constipation							
Pain							
Fatigue							
Tingling in fingers/toes							
Depression							

Personal notes:

—————————————————————————————

43

Week of: _____

Symptoms and side effects tracking

| 0 | 1 2 | 3 4 5 | 6 7 8 | 9 10 |
| none | low | mild | medium | high |

Day/date ——— ——— ——— ——— ——— ——— ———

Nausea ——— ——— ——— ——— ——— ——— ———

Appetite loss ——— ——— ——— ——— ——— ——— ———

Diarrhea ——— ——— ——— ——— ——— ——— ———

Constipation ——— ——— ——— ——— ——— ——— ———

Pain ——— ——— ——— ——— ——— ——— ———

Fatigue ——— ——— ——— ——— ——— ——— ———

Tingling in
fingers/toes ——— ——— ——— ——— ——— ——— ———

Depression ——— ——— ——— ——— ——— ——— ———

——— ——— ——— ——— ——— ——— ———

——— ——— ——— ——— ——— ——— ———

——— ——— ——— ——— ——— ——— ———

Personal notes:

Week of: _____

_____

_____

_____

Symptoms and side effects tracking

0	1 2	3 4 5	6 7 8	9 10
none	low	mild	medium	high

Day/date ——— ——— ——— ——— ——— ——— ———

Nausea ——— ——— ——— ——— ——— ——— ———

Appetite loss ——— ——— ——— ——— ——— ——— ———

Diarrhea ——— ——— ——— ——— ——— ——— ———

Constipation ——— ——— ——— ——— ——— ——— ———

Pain ——— ——— ——— ——— ——— ——— ———

Fatigue ——— ——— ——— ——— ——— ——— ———

Tingling in ——— ——— ——— ——— ——— ——— ———
fingers/toes

Depression ——— ——— ——— ——— ——— ——— ———

——————— ——— ——— ——— ——— ——— ———

——————— ——— ——— ——— ——— ——— ———

——————— ——— ——— ——— ——— ——— ———

Personal notes:

Week of: _____

Symptoms and side effects tracking

0	1 2	3 4 5	6 7 8	9 10
none	low	mild	medium	high

Day/date ——— ——— ——— ——— ——— ——— ———

Nausea ——— ——— ——— ——— ——— ——— ———

Appetite loss ——— ——— ——— ——— ——— ——— ———

Diarrhea ——— ——— ——— ——— ——— ——— ———

Constipation ——— ——— ——— ——— ——— ——— ———

Pain ——— ——— ——— ——— ——— ——— ———

Fatigue ——— ——— ——— ——— ——— ——— ———

Tingling in fingers/toes ——— ——— ——— ——— ——— ——— ———

Depression ——— ——— ——— ——— ——— ——— ———

——— ——— ——— ——— ——— ——— ——— ———

——— ——— ——— ——— ——— ——— ——— ———

——— ——— ——— ——— ——— ——— ——— ———

Personal notes:

Week of: _____

Symptoms and side effects tracking

	0	1 2	3 4 5	6 7 8	9 10
	none	low	mild	medium	high

Day/date	___	___	___	___	___	___	___
Nausea	___	___	___	___	___	___	___
Appetite loss	___	___	___	___	___	___	___
Diarrhea	___	___	___	___	___	___	___
Constipation	___	___	___	___	___	___	___
Pain	___	___	___	___	___	___	___
Fatigue	___	___	___	___	___	___	___
Tingling in fingers/toes	___	___	___	___	___	___	___
Depression	___	___	___	___	___	___	___
	___	___	___	___	___	___	___
	___	___	___	___	___	___	___
	___	___	___	___	___	___	___

Personal notes:

Week of:

Symptoms and side effects tracking

	0	1 2	3 4 5	6 7 8	9 10
	none	low	mild	medium	high

Day/date ——— ——— ——— ——— ——— ——— ———

Nausea

Appetite loss

Diarrhea

Constipation

Pain

Fatigue

Tingling in
fingers/toes

Depression

Personal notes:

Week of:

Symptoms and side effects tracking

Day/date ——— ——— ——— ——— ——— ——— ———

Nausea

Appetite loss

Diarrhea

Constipation

Pain

Fatigue

Tingling in
fingers/toes

Depression

Personal notes:

Week of: _____

Symptoms and side effects tracking

0	1 2	3 4 5	6 7 8	9 10
none	low	mild	medium	high

Day/date _____ _____ _____ _____ _____ _____ _____

Nausea

Appetite loss

Diarrhea

Constipation

Pain

Fatigue

Tingling in
fingers/toes

Depression

_____

_____

_____

Personal notes:

Week of: _____

Symptoms and side effects tracking

0	1 2	3 4 5	6 7 8	9 10
none	low	mild	medium	high

Day/date ——— ——— ——— ——— ——— ——— ———

Nausea

Appetite loss

Diarrhea

Constipation

Pain

Fatigue

Tingling in
fingers/toes

Depression

_____

_____

_____

Personal notes:

Week of: _____

Symptoms and side effects tracking

Day/date						
Nausea						
Appetite loss						
Diarrhea						
Constipation						
Pain						
Fatigue						
Tingling in fingers/toes						
Depression						

Personal notes:

Week of: _____

Symptoms and side effects tracking

0	1 2	3 4 5	6 7 8	9 10
none	low	mild	medium	high

Day/date ——— ——— ——— ——— ——— ——— ———

Nausea ——— ——— ——— ——— ——— ——— ———

Appetite loss ——— ——— ——— ——— ——— ——— ———

Diarrhea ——— ——— ——— ——— ——— ——— ———

Constipation ——— ——— ——— ——— ——— ——— ———

Pain ——— ——— ——— ——— ——— ——— ———

Fatigue ——— ——— ——— ——— ——— ——— ———

Tingling in ——— ——— ——— ——— ——— ——— ———
fingers/toes

Depression ——— ——— ——— ——— ——— ——— ———

_____ ——— ——— ——— ——— ——— ——— ———

_____ ——— ——— ——— ——— ——— ——— ———

_____ ——— ——— ——— ——— ——— ——— ———

Personal notes:

_____

_____

_____

_____

_____

_____

_____

_____

Week of:

Symptoms and side effects tracking

Day/date	——	——	——	——	——	——	——
Nausea	——	——	——	——	——	——	——
Appetite loss	——	——	——	——	——	——	——
Diarrhea	——	——	——	——	——	——	——
Constipation	——	——	——	——	——	——	——
Pain	——	——	——	——	——	——	——
Fatigue	——	——	——	——	——	——	——
Tingling in fingers/toes	——	——	——	——	——	——	——
Depression	——	——	——	——	——	——	——
————	——	——	——	——	——	——	——
————	——	——	——	——	——	——	——
————	——	——	——	——	——	——	——

Personal notes:

Week of: _____

Symptoms and side effects tracking

	0	1 2	3 4 5	6 7 8	9 10
	none	low	mild	medium	high

Day/date	———	———	———	———	———	———	———
Nausea	———	———	———	———	———	———	———
Appetite loss	———	———	———	———	———	———	———
Diarrhea	———	———	———	———	———	———	———
Constipation	———	———	———	———	———	———	———
Pain	———	———	———	———	———	———	———
Fatigue	———	———	———	———	———	———	———
Tingling in fingers/toes	———	———	———	———	———	———	———
Depression	———	———	———	———	———	———	———
———————	———	———	———	———	———	———	———
———————	———	———	———	———	———	———	———
———————	———	———	———	———	———	———	———

Personal notes:

Week of:

Symptoms and side effects tracking

0	1 2	3 4 5	6 7 8	9 10
none	low	mild	medium	high

Day/date ——— ——— ——— ——— ——— ——— ———

Nausea ——— ——— ——— ——— ——— ——— ———

Appetite loss ——— ——— ——— ——— ——— ——— ———

Diarrhea ——— ——— ——— ——— ——— ——— ———

Constipation ——— ——— ——— ——— ——— ——— ———

Pain ——— ——— ——— ——— ——— ——— ———

Fatigue ——— ——— ——— ——— ——— ——— ———

Tingling in ——— ——— ——— ——— ——— ——— ———
fingers/toes

Depression ——— ——— ——— ——— ——— ——— ———

——— ——— ——— ——— ——— ——— ——— ———

——— ——— ——— ——— ——— ——— ——— ———

——— ——— ——— ——— ——— ——— ——— ———

Personal notes:

_____

_____

_____

_____

_____

_____

_____

_____

Symptoms and side effects tracking

	0	1 2	3 4 5	6 7 8	9 10
	none	low	mild	medium	high

Day/date	——	——	——	——	——	——	——
Nausea	——	——	——	——	——	——	——
Appetite loss	——	——	——	——	——	——	——
Diarrhea	——	——	——	——	——	——	——
Constipation	——	——	——	——	——	——	——
Pain	——	——	——	——	——	——	——
Fatigue	——	——	——	——	——	——	——
Tingling in fingers/toes	——	——	——	——	——	——	——
Depression	——	——	——	——	——	——	——
	——	——	——	——	——	——	——
	——	——	——	——	——	——	——
	——	——	——	——	——	——	——

Personal notes:

Week of:

Symptoms and side effects tracking

	0	1 2	3 4 5	6 7 8	9 10
	none	low	mild	medium	high

Day/date ——— ——— ——— ——— ——— ———

Nausea						
Appetite loss						
Diarrhea						
Constipation						
Pain						
Fatigue						
Tingling in fingers/toes						
Depression						

Personal notes:

Week of: _____

Symptoms and side effects tracking

Day/date ——— ——— ——— ——— ——— ——— ———

Nausea

Appetite loss

Diarrhea

Constipation

Pain

Fatigue

Tingling in
fingers/toes

Depression

Personal notes:

Week of: _____

Symptoms and side effects tracking

0	1 2	3 4 5	6 7 8	9 10
none	low	mild	medium	high

Day/date	———	———	———	———	———	———	———
Nausea							
Appetite loss							
Diarrhea							
Constipation							
Pain							
Fatigue							
Tingling in fingers/toes							
Depression							

Personal notes:

Week of: _____

Symptoms and side effects tracking

Day/date ———   ———   ———   ———   ———   ———   ———

Nausea

Appetite loss

Diarrhea

Constipation

Pain

Fatigue

Tingling in
fingers/toes

Depression

Personal notes:

Week of:

Symptoms and side effects tracking

	0	1 2	3 4 5	6 7 8	9 10
	none	low	mild	medium	high

Day/date ——— ——— ——— ——— ——— ——— ———

Nausea							
Appetite loss							
Diarrhea							
Constipation							
Pain							
Fatigue							
Tingling in fingers/toes							
Depression							

Personal notes:

81

Symptoms and side effects tracking

0	1 2	3 4 5	6 7 8	9 10
none	low	mild	medium	high

Day/date ——— ——— ——— ——— ——— ——— ———

Nausea ——— ——— ——— ——— ——— ——— ———

Appetite loss ——— ——— ——— ——— ——— ——— ———

Diarrhea ——— ——— ——— ——— ——— ——— ———

Constipation ——— ——— ——— ——— ——— ——— ———

Pain ——— ——— ——— ——— ——— ——— ———

Fatigue ——— ——— ——— ——— ——— ——— ———

Tingling in ——— ——— ——— ——— ——— ——— ———
fingers/toes

Depression ——— ——— ——— ——— ——— ——— ———

——————— ——— ——— ——— ——— ——— ———

——————— ——— ——— ——— ——— ——— ———

——————— ——— ——— ——— ——— ——— ———

Personal notes:

Week of:

Symptoms and side effects tracking

Day/date							
Nausea							
Appetite loss							
Diarrhea							
Constipation							
Pain							
Fatigue							
Tingling in fingers/toes							
Depression							

Personal notes:

Symptoms and side effects tracking

0	1 2	3 4 5	6 7 8	9 10
none	low	mild	medium	high

Day/date ——— ——— ——— ——— ——— ——— ———

Nausea							
Appetite loss							
Diarrhea							
Constipation							
Pain							
Fatigue							
Tingling in fingers/toes							
Depression							

Personal notes:

Week of:

Symptoms and side effects tracking

	0	1 2	3 4 5	6 7 8	9 10
	none	low	mild	medium	high

Day/date ——— ——— ——— ——— ——— ——— ———

Nausea	——	——	——	——	——	——
Appetite loss	——	——	——	——	——	——
Diarrhea	——	——	——	——	——	——
Constipation	——	——	——	——	——	——
Pain	——	——	——	——	——	——
Fatigue	——	——	——	——	——	——
Tingling in fingers/toes	——	——	——	——	——	——
Depression	——	——	——	——	——	——
————	——	——	——	——	——	——
————	——	——	——	——	——	——
————	——	——	——	——	——	——

Personal notes:

Week of:

Symptoms and side effects tracking

0	1 2	3 4 5	6 7 8	9 10
none	low	mild	medium	high

Day/date	——	——	——	——	——	——	——
Nausea	——	——	——	——	——	——	——
Appetite loss	——	——	——	——	——	——	——
Diarrhea	——	——	——	——	——	——	——
Constipation	——	——	——	——	——	——	——
Pain	——	——	——	——	——	——	——
Fatigue	——	——	——	——	——	——	——
Tingling in fingers/toes	——	——	——	——	——	——	——
Depression	——	——	——	——	——	——	——
_____	——	——	——	——	——	——	——
_____	——	——	——	——	——	——	——
_____	——	——	——	——	——	——	——

Personal notes:

Week of:

Symptoms and side effects tracking

0	1 2	3 4 5	6 7 8	9 10
none	low	mild	medium	high

Day/date ——— ——— ——— ——— ——— ——— ———

Nausea

Appetite loss

Diarrhea

Constipation

Pain

Fatigue

Tingling in fingers/toes

Depression

Personal notes:

Being as prepared as possible can help you get the most out of each health care visit. To help you get prepared...

Review your calendars

Review your weekly and monthly calendars before each appointment. Take some time to look for information, questions or any trends in symptoms or side effects.

Get your questions ready

Between visits, try to keep a running list of questions you have. Then, as you go through your calendars, add to your list any questions you may have forgotten to write down, plus any new ones that come to mind. Once your list is complete, highlight the questions that are a priority for you to get answered.

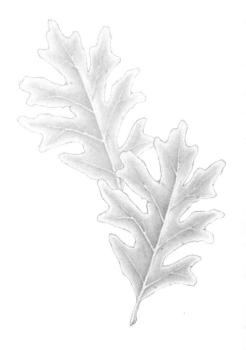

Discuss anything unusual

If you feel that something is unusual for you or if you see any trends developing, it is really important to share the information with your health care team, even if you think it may be unimportant. If anything impacts your life or how you are feeling, discuss it—you will not be seen as a nuisance.

The WriteTrack can help

You may find it helpful to use the following pages to keep track of appointments, questions, and information you want to discuss at each health care visit. You may even want to show this to your health care team to make sure you get all of the information you want. If you need additional space or if you want a more "portable" version to carry with you, make photocopies of these pages.

> *"Quality of life was a priority for our family. Tracking my husband's symptoms provided us with the information we needed to communicate his needs more effectively. There was so much to think about. Writing down our questions helped us remember what we wanted to ask and allowed us to make better use of our time during health care visits."*
>
> Peggy Wiederholt

Appointment date_____ Time_____

Your usual weight_____

Your weight this visit_____

Questions/issues to discuss with your health care team

_____

_____

_____

_____

_____

_____

_____

_____

_____

_____

_____

_____

_____

_____

_____

_____

_____

_____

_____

_____

_____

_____

Record any trends you have noticed relating to symptoms and side effects

Nausea _____

_____

Appetite loss _____

_____

Diarrhea _____

_____

Constipation _____

_____

Pain _____

_____

Fatigue _____

_____

Tingling in
fingers/toes _____

_____

Depression _____

_____

_____

_____

_____

Appointment date_____ Time_____

Your usual weight_____

Your weight this visit_____

Questions/issues to discuss with your health care team

_____

_____

_____

_____

_____

_____

_____

_____

_____

_____

_____

_____

_____

_____

_____

_____

_____

_____

_____

_____

_____

Record any trends you have noticed relating to symptoms and side effects

Nausea _____

_____

Appetite loss _____

_____

Diarrhea _____

_____

Constipation _____

_____

Pain _____

_____

Fatigue _____

_____

Tingling in
fingers/toes _____

_____

Depression _____

_____

_____

_____

_____

_____

Appointment date_____ Time_____

Your usual weight_____

Your weight this visit_____

Questions/issues to discuss with your health care team

_____
_____
_____
_____
_____
_____
_____
_____
_____
_____
_____
_____
_____
_____
_____
_____
_____
_____
_____
_____
_____

Record any trends you have noticed relating to symptoms and side effects

Nausea _____

_____

Appetite loss _____

_____

Diarrhea _____

_____

Constipation _____

_____

Pain _____

_____

Fatigue _____

_____

Tingling in _____
fingers/toes

_____

Depression _____

_____

_____

_____

_____

Appointment date_____ Time_____

Your usual weight_____

Your weight this visit_____

Questions/issues to discuss with your health care team

Record any trends you have noticed relating to symptoms and side effects

Nausea _____

_____

Appetite loss _____

_____

Diarrhea _____

_____

Constipation _____

_____

Pain _____

_____

Fatigue _____

_____

Tingling in
fingers/toes _____

_____

Depression _____

_____

_____

_____

_____

_____

Appointment date_____ Time_____

Your usual weight_____

Your weight this visit_____

Questions/issues to discuss with your health care team

Record any trends you have noticed relating to symptoms and side effects

Nausea _____

_____

Appetite loss _____

_____

Diarrhea _____

_____

Constipation _____

_____

Pain _____

_____

Fatigue _____

_____

Tingling in
fingers/toes _____

_____

Depression _____

_____

_____ _____

_____

_____ _____

_____

Appointment date_____ Time_____

Your usual weight_____

Your weight this visit_____

Questions/issues to discuss with your health care team

Record any trends you have noticed relating to symptoms and side effects

Nausea _____

_____

Appetite loss _____

_____

Diarrhea _____

_____

Constipation _____

_____

Pain _____

_____

Fatigue _____

_____

Tingling in _____
fingers/toes

Depression _____

_____

_____

_____

_____

_____

Appointment date_____ Time_____

Your usual weight_____

Your weight this visit_____

Questions/issues to discuss with your health care team

Record any trends you have noticed relating to symptoms and side effects

Nausea _____

_____

Appetite loss _____

_____

Diarrhea _____

_____

Constipation _____

_____

Pain _____

_____

Fatigue _____

_____

Tingling in
fingers/toes _____

_____

Depression _____

_____

_____

_____

_____

Appointment date_____ Time_____

Your usual weight_____

Your weight this visit_____

Questions/issues to discuss with your health care team

Record any trends you have noticed relating to symptoms and side effects

Nausea _____

_____

Appetite loss _____

_____

Diarrhea _____

_____

Constipation _____

_____

Pain _____

_____

Fatigue _____

_____

Tingling in
fingers/toes _____

_____

Depression _____

_____

_____

_____

_____

_____

Appointment date_____ Time_____

Your usual weight_____

Your weight this visit_____

Questions/issues to discuss with your health care team

_____

_____

_____

_____

_____

_____

_____

_____

_____

_____

_____

_____

_____

_____

_____

_____

_____

_____

_____

_____

Record any trends you have noticed relating to symptoms and side effects

Nausea

Appetite loss

Diarrhea

Constipation

Pain

Fatigue

Tingling in fingers/toes

Depression

Appointment date_____ Time_____

Your usual weight_____

Your weight this visit_____

Questions/issues to discuss with your health care team

Record any trends you have noticed relating to symptoms and side effects

Nausea

_____

_____

Appetite loss

_____

_____

Diarrhea

_____

_____

Constipation

_____

_____

Pain

_____

_____

Fatigue

_____

_____

Tingling in
fingers/toes

_____

Depression

_____

_____

_____

_____

_____

_____

Appointment date_____ Time_____

Your usual weight_____

Your weight this visit_____

Questions/issues to discuss with your health care team

Record any trends you have noticed relating to symptoms and side effects

Nausea _____

_____

Appetite loss _____

_____

Diarrhea _____

_____

Constipation _____

_____

Pain _____

_____

Fatigue _____

_____

Tingling in fingers/toes _____

_____

Depression _____

_____

_____ _____

_____

_____ _____

_____

Appointment date_____ Time_____

Your usual weight_____

Your weight this visit_____

Questions/issues to discuss with your health care team

Record any trends you have noticed relating to symptoms and side effects

Nausea _____

_____

Appetite loss _____

_____

Diarrhea _____

_____

Constipation _____

_____

Pain _____

_____

Fatigue _____

_____

Tingling in
fingers/toes _____

_____

Depression _____

_____

_____

_____

_____

_____

MEDICINES

Throughout treatment for cancer, you will probably be taking different medicines. You may want to use these pages to help you keep track of medicines prescribed by your health care team, as well as any over-the-counter medicines or vitamins you take.

If you have any questions or concerns about your medicines, talk to your health care team. If something is unclear, ask for another explanation. Keep in mind that your pharmacist is an expert in medicines and can also answer any questions you have.

Name of medicine	Purpose	Date medicine started

Always take your medicine exactly as instructed by your health care team. Before making any changes in the amount of medicine you take or when you take it, talk to your health care team. Also talk to your health care team before you stop taking any medicine.

Dose how much/how often	Date medicine stopped	Notes

MEDICINES

Name of medicine	Purpose	Date medicine started

MEDICINES

Dose how much/how often	Date medicine stopped	Notes

Good nutrition is an important part of daily living. It helps you to maintain strength and have a better quality of life. Chemotherapy, radiation therapy, or the cancer itself may make eating and drinking difficult. Ask your health care team for guidelines on what types of food and beverages you should eat and drink and what you should avoid.

If you are having problems eating or drinking, your health care team may have some helpful suggestions. You may want to use these pages to record information about your diet. Keep in mind that your nutrition needs may change.

Recommended Diet:

_____

_____

_____

_____

_____

_____

_____

_____

_____

_____

_____

_____

_____

_____

_____

_____

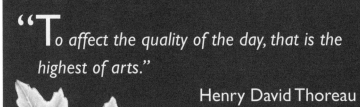

"*To affect the quality of the day, that is the highest of arts.*"

Henry David Thoreau

Other Helpful Suggestions:

Things to Avoid:

Throughout treatment for cancer, many people found it useful to keep track of laboratory tests. While tracking laboratory tests is not for everyone, you may find it helpful. By reviewing the different tests and results, you can look for certain trends that may be developing. To help keep track of this information, ask for photocopies of all your lab tests and keep them in a file or envelope.

You can also use these pages to record other tests and results. Write each test you want to track in the chart. If you have any questions about what the results mean or if the results differ from previous tests, talk to your health care team.

Name of test	Purpose	Date	Results/blood counts

Name of test	Purpose	Date	Results/blood counts

Name of test	Purpose	Date	Results/blood counts

Name of test	Purpose	Date	Results/blood counts

One of the more daunting tasks while going through treatment for cancer is dealing with medical bills and health insurance. It may sometimes feel as if you are facing "mountains" of paperwork. Sometimes the paperwork can be difficult to understand or figure out, so it is important to be organized in a way that will help you stay on top of it.

Keep accurate records

Accurate record keeping will make it easy for you to find information if there are any questions about payments and insurance coverage. Keep copies of all medical bills, insurance statements (also called Explanation of Benefits), receipts, and any letters or correspondence with your health care team and insurance provider. In some cases, medical expenses may be tax deductible, so you may need these records and receipts when your income tax is prepared.

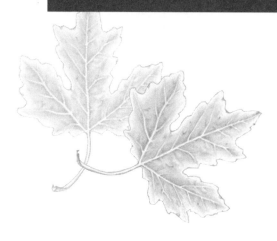

"Patience and perserverance have a magical effect before which difficulties disappear and obstacles vanish."

John Quincy Adams

The WriteTrack can help

If you think it will help you to track your medical bills and health insurance, *The WriteTrack* can help you get organized and keep accurate records...

cs Record all dates that treatments, procedures or lab tests are performed in the weekly and monthly calendars. This information can be used to cross reference bills and insurance statements.

cs Keep the name of your health insurance provider along with the plan, group number, and a summary of your plan benefits in a handy place. Record this information on the pages that follow or in the Important Telephone Numbers section of *The WriteTrack* (see pages 160-161).

cs Document all telephone conversations with your health insurance provider on the following pages. Write the date and time of each conversation in case you need to recall information or retrace certain events. Health insurance providers often record phone calls — they may be able to go back and listen to the conversation if needed.

cs Record your mileage and travel expenses to and from treatments and health care visits in your weekly calendar—they may be tax deductible.

Set up a filing system

cs Ask a family member or friend to help you organize and keep track of your medical bills and health insurance claims.

cs Keep copies of all insurance forms, claims, statements, and correspondence.

cs Write the date at the top of each document you receive.

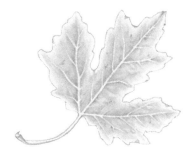

Medical bills and health insurance telephone log

Your health insurance provider _____

Plan/identification number(s) _____

_____

Telephone number _____

Date/time	Reason for call	Who you talked to

Phone extension	Notes

> "**A**sking for help was so hard, but I soon learned it gave me many gifts. I got things done... it helped me save energy...and more important, I got to see a side of my family and friends I never saw before. They also got to see a new side of me. Asking for help brought me closer to my family and friends."
>
> Sue
> *Ovarian Cancer Survivor*

As you go through treatment, getting support from family and friends can be very important. It may not be easy for you to ask for support, especially if you are usually an independent person, but keep in mind that family and friends will want to be there for you—to offer support and help you when you need it most. Also remember that family and friends may not be sure about the type of support you will want and how they can help you.

When asking for help, try to give family and friends specific ways to help or things to do. This can often be a source of relief to you and them. By asking for help, you will get the things you need done and you can strengthen relationships. Family and friends will also feel useful and they may find it easier to talk to you about your cancer, your treatment, and how both of you are feeling.

How to ask family and friends for support

Delegating responsibilities and asking for help can sometimes be difficult, but once you start, it can make getting through treatment more manageable. Here are some tips for getting the support you need...

- Make a list of all the things you could really use help with. Maybe it's house cleaning, transportation, making meals, walking the dog, taking children to school and after-school activities, shopping, and running errands.

- Identify someone who has offered to help you or someone you would feel comfortable asking for help.

- Be straightforward when asking for help.

- Give the person helping you a timeline to work with—that way you will both know what is needed and when it's needed.

"*When I was going through my treatments, my friends and family kept asking 'How can I help?' I wasn't used to asking for help...it took me a while to think of ways they could help me. What I really needed was to have someone come over to play basketball with my son on Saturdays... that really helped me and him.*"

Lou
Lung Cancer Survivor

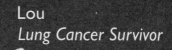

"Throughout my cancer treatments, my doctors, family, and friends were really supportive...but they could never really understand what I was going through. Sometimes I felt so alone and isolated. Joining a support group gave me a chance to express my feelings... I could finally connect with others who knew exactly what I was going through."

Jill
Breast Cancer Survivor

Many people with cancer find it very helpful to talk to and get support from others who have been through diagnosis and treatment. In fact, people often find they get some of the best information and helpful tips from others with firsthand experience.

One way to do this is to become involved with a support group. Support groups provide an ideal forum for talking about the range of emotions and feelings you have and sharing your experiences, issues, concerns, fears, and even the good things that are happening to you. By drawing on the strength and experiences of others, you can gain a sense of confidence...you may even find humor and lighthearted moments in hearing some of the stories from other group members.

Different support groups have different personalities...and we all have different needs. You might want to try a few support groups, until you find one you are comfortable with.

Reaching out for support is a personal decision. You may choose to participate in a support group, then again, they may not interest you. Instead, you may want to consider individual or family counseling. The choice is yours—just know that different types of support are available if you want or need to take advantage of them.

How to find a support group

❧ You may find an "informal" support group develops between you and others in the waiting room or suites of the cancer unit where you get treatment.

❧ Ask your health care team — especially your social worker or oncology nurse about support groups.

❧ Call the American Cancer Society at 800-ACS-2345. This will link you directly to your local chapter of the American Cancer Society where you can find out about support groups in your area.

❧ Ask about ongoing support groups at local churches or with religious organizations in your area.

❧ Consider organizing your own support group with friends and acquaintances who are undergoing treatment for cancer.

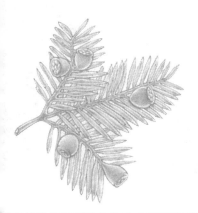

Valuable resources for support

Cancer Care, Inc.
The Cancer Care Counseling Line

Cancer Care is a social agency that provides direct help (counseling, educational programs, and referrals) to patients and families as they cope with emotional, financial, psychological, and other aspects of cancer and its treatment. A toll-free counseling line can connect you or a family member with a professional Cancer Care social worker.

800-813-HOPE (800-813-4673)

The Group Room™

The Group Room is the only call-in talk radio support group for people dealing with cancer, their families, friends, and health care providers. Call for information.

800-GRP-ROOM (800-477-7666)

National Coalition for Cancer Survivorship (NCCS)

NCCS is a network of independent organizations and individuals that act as advocates for cancer survivors and offer referrals to local services. Call the NCCS Response Line, leave your name and address, and information will be mailed to you.

888-YES-NCCS (888-937-6227)

A cancer diagnosis can be overwhelming for you, your family and friends. It can also affect your relationships with others. While loved ones can provide much needed support, sometimes communication may be more difficult due to anxiety and fear.

People often say that dealing with cancer is like being on an emotional roller coaster. Feelings vary from person-to-person and minute-to-minute. Your loved ones may not know what to say for fear of saying the wrong thing. Some relationships grow stronger while others can drift apart. Depression is common among cancer patients.

While some people are able to work through their feelings, others find it helpful to meet with a social worker or health psychologist. Remember that your emotional well-being is as important as your physical health.

Sexuality greatly affects how you feel about yourself and how you relate to others. Concern about body image and the effects of cancer treatments on sexual performance and fertility are important quality of life issues. Don't be afraid or embarrassed to talk about these concerns with your health care team. For more information on fertility, contact fertileHOPE at 1-888-994-HOPE or www.fertilehope.org.

"When I was diagnosed with breast cancer at the age of 30, I was concerned about how I could go through treatment and still be able to have a family. I found peace by working closely with my physicians and a genetic counselor. They helped me understand my options so I could make an informed decision about my treatment and my future."

Michele
Breast Cancer Survivor

FAITH AND SPIRITUALITY

Faith and spirituality are an important part of many people's lives. This may be especially true for someone diagnosed with cancer. If you have a religious belief, you may find strength and comfort through prayer or you may suddenly question your faith because of what is happening to you. Whatever you are feeling, you may find it helpful to talk with a religious leader, spiritual advisor or counselor.

You may not have an affiliation with a religion, but may have certain values and beliefs that guide your daily living. Talking to others who share your beliefs may help you cope with your cancer.

"Faith provided our family with an inner strength that we never imagined we possessed. We prayed together often and found that it helped us to face every challenge with courage and dignity."

Peggy Wiederholt

COMPLIMENTARY, ALTERNATIVE AND INTEGRATIVE MEDICINE

The terms used to describe different approaches to medical treatment can be confusing.

Conventional medicine refers to standard medicine as practiced by physicians in the United States. Conventional treatments have been scientifically researched for safety and effectiveness.

Complimentary and Alternative medicine are medical practices, therapies and products that are not considered part of conventional medicine. **Complimentary** medicine is used *together with* conventional medicine. **Alternative** medicine is used *in place of* conventional medicine.

Integrative medicine *combines* conventional medical therapies and complimentary/alternative therapies for which there is some scientific evidence that they are safe and effective.

The National Center for Complimentary and Alternative Medicine (NCCAM) is a component of the National Institutes of Health (NIH). NCCAM can provide you with information on which complimentary and alternative therapies work, which do not, and why. If you have questions or would like more information about complimentary and alternative medicine, you may contact:

NCCAM Clearinghouse
Toll free: 1-888-644-6226
E-mail: info@nccam.nih.gov
Web site: nccam.nih.gov

Evaluating Web Sites

Many people use the Web to find information about treatment options for their cancer. While some of these sites are a valuable resource, others may have information that is confusing or misleading.

Refer to the NCCAM Web site for...
"10 Things to Know
About Evaluating Medical
Resources on the Web"

Palliative care

Palliative care services are available at many medical centers. The aims of palliative care are to meet the physical, emotional and spiritual needs of people with serious illness, and the needs of their families and loved ones.

The palliative care team members include physicians, nurses, pharmacists, social workers, psychologists and chaplains. Depending upon your needs, a team member may be involved in your care for a short time or as part of long-term care. This may include care provided in your home.

Palliative care provides compassionate "comfort care" to achieve the best quality of life for patients and their loved ones. Services include managing pain and symptoms, providing support to patients and families, and helping families and friends in their roles as caregivers. Hospice is an organizaton that provides palliative care for people with a terminal illness or injury.

If this is something that you think would be helpful, ask your health care team about palliative care services in your area.

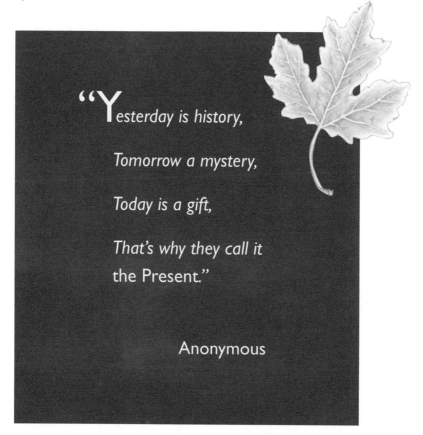

"Yesterday is history,

Tomorrow a mystery,

Today is a gift,

That's why they call it
the Present."

Anonymous

Using the Monthly Calendars

On the pages that follow, you will find blank calendars you can use to help you see the bigger picture—that is, what is happening each month as you go through treatment.

To get started using the monthly calendars, write in the name of the month at the top of each page. Then write in the correct dates that correspond with the days of that month. Use the calendars as you choose—you may want to use them to help you keep track of appointments with your health care team, dates and times of treatments, business meetings, and personal events such as birthdays and anniversaries. The most important thing is for you to use the monthly calendars in the way that best meets your needs.

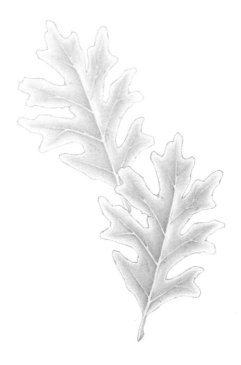

MONTH: _____

Monday	Tuesday	Wednesday
____	____	____
____	____	____
____	____	____
____	____	____
____	____	____

Thursday	Friday	Saturday/Sunday
———	———	———
———	———	———
———	———	———
———	———	———
———	———	———

Month:

Monday	Tuesday	Wednesday
____	____	____
____	____	____
____	____	____
____	____	____
____		____

Thursday	Friday	Saturday/Sunday
___	___	___
___	___	___
___	___	___
___	___	___
___	___	___

Month: _____

Monday	Tuesday	Wednesday
___	___	___
___	___	___
___	___	___
___	___	___
___	___	___

Thursday	Friday	Saturday/Sunday
___	___	___
___	___	___
___	___	___
___	___	___
___	___	___

MONTH: _____

Monday	Tuesday	Wednesday
____	____	____
____	____	____
____	____	____
____	____	____
____	____	____

Thursday	Friday	Saturday/Sunday
————	————	————
————	————	————
————	————	————
————	————	————
————	————	————

Month: _____

Monday	Tuesday	Wednesday
———	———	———
———	———	———
———	———	———
———	———	———
———	———	———

Thursday	Friday	Saturday/Sunday
___	___	___
___	___	___
___	___	___
___	___	___
___	___	___

Month:

Monday	Tuesday	Wednesday
___	___	___
___	___	___
___	___	___
___	___	___
___	___	___

Thursday	Friday	Saturday/Sunday
———	———	———
———	———	———
———	———	———
———	———	———
———	———	———

Month:

Monday	Tuesday	Wednesday
____	____	____
____	____	____
____	____	____
____	____	____
____	____	____

Thursday	Friday	Saturday/Sunday
___	___	___
___	___	___
___	___	___
___	___	___
___	___	___

Month: _____

Monday	Tuesday	Wednesday
___	___	___
___	___	___
___	___	___
___	___	___
___	___	___

Thursday	Friday	Saturday/Sunday
——	——	——
——	——	——
——	——	——
——	——	——
——	——	——

IMPORTANT TELEPHONE NUMBERS

The WriteTrack includes a number of valuable resources to help as you cope with cancer and its treatment. In addition to the services already described in *The WriteTrack*, these organizations can also refer you to other organizations that specialize in providing information and services for specific types of cancer.

Quick reference to valuable resources

American Cancer Society (ACS)..800-ACS-2345

Cancer Care Counseling Line..800-813-HOPE

National Cancer Institute (NCI) 800-4-CANCER

National Coalition for Cancer Survivorship (NCCS)......................888-YES-NCCS

Your health insurance

Provider

Telephone number

Plan/identification number(s)

Your health care team

Name	Their role	Telephone number

Name   **Telephone number**

"Throughout the years of your life you will face many challenges, remember that you can climb the highest mountain, drive through the roughest storm, soar across the bluest sky, or even sail across the roughest waters. It is only destined by your attitude where you will end up in life."

Angela Duvall

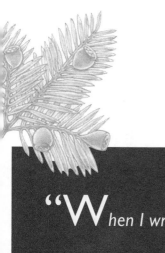

"**W**hen I write, I can shake off all of my cares."

Anne Frank

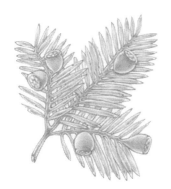

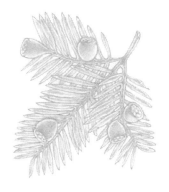

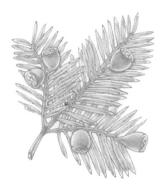

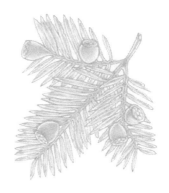

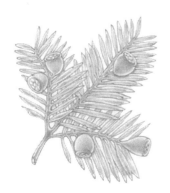

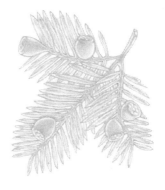

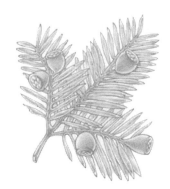

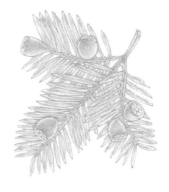

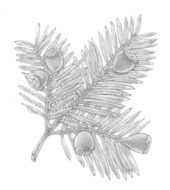

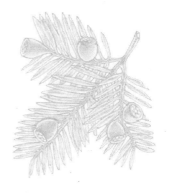

"I wanted a perfect ending. Now I've learned the hard way, that some poems don't rhyme, and some stories don't have a clear beginning, middle and end. Life is about not knowing, having to change, taking a moment and making the best of it, without knowing what's going to happen next."

Gilda Radner